I Wanted It

*A step-by-step
weight loss guide
for the business traveler*

by Caryn Gillen

Advanced Praise

"I don't travel much anymore but I still found Caryn Gillen's protocol for sensible weight loss very valuable. Her plan is not really about food or willpower. The tools she shares go way deeper. She gets at the ultimate truth, as she puts it, that weight is most fundamentally an excuse for ducking out of your life.

Caryn writes with engaging authenticity that draws you in and makes you really want to succeed - no matter how many times you've failed at weight loss before. If you are sick of obsessing about weight and food, this book will change your life."

-Margie King

"This book is written so it feels like a personal experience for every reader. It is written in a way that feels like the author is working with you directly. Not only is it motivational but it is also a quick read so you can get started with seeing the results you want. Definitely a book worth reading!"

-Gina Meucci

"One of my favorite ways to spend a Sunday afternoon is reading a diet book while eating a whole package of cookies. You can feel virtuous about reading the book and still enjoy yourself. When I began reading Gillen's I Wanted It, I didn't even bother with the cookies because it was short. It was an easy read without all the padding that most diet books include to get up to 300 pages. And it was concrete and informative. I tend to read things and think, "That's a good idea," and then immediately forget them, but I Wanted It includes worksheets and lists to remind you of the important points. Finally, her program is very do-able. I kept reading and thinking, "I can do that." I'm very excited about trying Gillen's program as soon as I go shopping and buy some healthy food. This could be a life-changer for anyone who has struggled with food in the past."

-Carrie Enge

"Caryn's book is tried and true--not rocket science but rather, reality and clarity wrapped in a palatable dose of do-ability."

- Shoo Salasky

"My favorite part of this book is that I already have everything I need to make the system work for me. It's very frustrating to be told I need to buy specific products in order to achieve weight loss, that's what's mostly out there, and what I've tried previously. I'll admit, some of the things you mention turned me off - I don't enjoy salad and being told I can't eat something pushes me toward it, I'm a rebel! However, reading the book in its entirety gave me well rounded perspective to better understand the ideology and I'm going to put some of these things into practice right away."
        -Jackie Jamison

"This book is a real world perspective on how our bodies treat food. Knowing that eating several small meals is what's keeping our bodies from working efficiently and how much sugar negatively affects the body was great information. I feel much better now that I've shifted my eating habits and don't look at food as something more than the fuel I need to live. Great read!!"
        -Connie Ellis

"I'm writing this review because I love reading people's real experiences before I dive into trying something new or different, I hands down recommend this book! I had thought of myself as a healthy eater and I was trying to be more active but had kinda hit a spot where I wasn't getting anywhere and not meeting goals I set for myself. I read this book and did the coaching with the author and started to see results and learning more about myself and my body in the process, there are some key phrases in this book like "show up for yourself" I tell myself that everyday now and live by it, I need to take care of myself like I take care of others! I think the book is amazing and I would recommend it to anyone wanting to better themselves and make a lifestyle change but the coaching takes it to another level, having someone that is passionate about your success and helping meet goals you never thought were possible is priceless..."

-Karen Hammers

"Caryn is one of the best weight loss coaches I know. Having read her book and being both a Life Coach and Psychotherapist, I'm insisting that any client of mine needing to lose weight, be it 10 or 100 pounds, buy her book ASAP. Her book lays things out in clear and uncomplicated terms. Caryn distills things down into the clearest and easiest to understand terms, which is exactly how she coaches people. Clean, Clear and straight to the point. If you want to loose weight, get this book and follow the directions. You WILL lose the weight."

    -Veronique Vaillancourt LCSW

x

Foreword

I met Caryn several years ago when we found ourselves on the same journey to find a sustainable way of eating healthy and losing weight. As busy Moms and Professionals we had a long list of "to dos" and losing weight was always at the top but never seemed to get done. Crazy expectations and what feels like a chronic shortage of time mean everyone else's needs get taken care of first. Early on, many of our conversations revolved around how to find balance without using food as a coping mechanism. Since using the tools Caryn outlines in her book to get to goal weight, we have been able to spend our time together brainstorming about writing, talking about helping clients and patients lose weight, and even go stand up paddle boarding on Lake Tahoe. Having a food protocol makes such a difference in freeing up time to pursue your true passion.

What was a physician doing looking for a new way to eat when counseling patients on nutrition is part of my job? I had to get past the medical dogma that preaches, "Just eat less, low-fat of course, and exercise more!" The eat-less strategy occasionally works, but when it does it's as much to my surprise as anyone else's. It's not that doctors actually want patients to fail, but we haven't been trained in alternatives that actually work. There isn't any secret pill or method we save for ourselves. Also, like many other women, I am practicing in a profession that while focused on the service of others, forgot to teach me to leave time for taking care of myself.

Whether you spend the majority of your work life traveling or find yourself out of town just occasionally, you still have to negotiate obstacles like crack-of-dawn meetings, 5-minute lunches – if they happen at all – and no-notice schedule changes that completely disrupt normal routines. As a young doctor in training, the distance I traveled was only 3.7 miles to work, but every fourth day I spent over 30 consecutive hours inside the hospital tethered to instant notification by 1, 2, or 3 pagers. With very little control over my personal schedule, let alone my eating (grab it when you can), the box of warm donuts on the staffing room table each morning at 7a.m. seemed like a small, but necessary escape. Honestly, they trained us to do almost anything for food, especially pizza. As an attending (a practicing and fully-licensed physician) I am no longer confined to the hospital but I still spend fully 25% of my life attached to patients through a pager – ready to drop everything no matter whether I'm sleeping, in the shower, or about to sit down to a meal with the family. That feeling of needing to be rewarded for extraordinary service is common to both my on-call routine and business travel. The meals now are usually served in nice restaurants instead of cardboard boxes, but the message is still the same – you deserve this because you work so hard!

What a unique perspective Caryn presents, that work isn't something to be endured but an opportunity to return to our personal lives energized and healthier than when we first set off. Instead of needing a reward, we get what we actually deserve: Our lives back.

Caryn's interest in helping people pursue their goals for change is both professional and personal. Her enthusiasm for coaching clients is evident at all times. She's studied this, she's lived it, and she's taught it to others through her coaching practice. She sees it as her true life's work to help women achieve their weight loss goals and end the STRUGGLE. Her direct, no nonsense approach means that if you are working with her, things are going to get done! In medicine and with proven success, we use physical therapists and mental health counselors regularly as part of treatment plans for chronic diseases. Weight loss coaches and life coaches have the same meaningful value in helping patients achieve their healthcare goals. Fifteen minutes is just not enough time for me to help a family set a weight loss goal, teach them the key principles of nutrition, demonstrate effective tools, and most importantly prepare them to deal with the mental challenges involved in making the whole process work. But it *is* enough time to create an effective team to help them get started on their goal.

My specialty is pediatrics. I wish obesity weren't something I spent a lot of time treating but it is the number one thing I spend time on that I was never trained during residency to do. And usually, it isn't just the child I need to treat, but the family as well. Caryn is 'spot on' when she talks about how she was worried her struggle with food had the potential to spill over to her daughter. The behaviors we model for our children are much more powerful than any lecture or advice we share with them. After all, they love us. We need to learn to love ourselves.

I promise you nothing bad will happen to you if you follow the recommendation in this book to eliminate flour and sugar. Nothing bad will happen to your children either! What I can guarantee from personal experience is that you won't be as hungry as you were on a low-fat diet and that means sustainability, which is the best predictor of maintaining weight loss. Food in its wild state (close to the way it came out of nature) isn't sexy, doesn't have a high profit margin, and doesn't scream SNACK but it is the fuel your body appreciates. Your children may complain (temporarily!) about the lack of cheesy fishy snack crackers but those crackers are no more appropriate fuel for them than they are for your car.

Food journals and planning ahead both have great data to recommend them as part of your weight loss tool kit. As Caryn points out, when we work/travel we fall into routines. With efficient (even 5 minutes) planning ahead of time you can take advantage of that fact with your new protocol; achieving the result you actually wanted. Get paid to lose weight! Fasting is definitely worth considering if you are an adult who is not taking any medications that affect your blood sugar. I fast once a week to help with my weight loss, improve my insulin sensitivity, refocus my eating goals for the week, and decrease my chance of developing Alzheimer's disease. I think it's important to recognize that a diet that emphasizes eating ready-made snacks all day has only been around for the last few decades. Our bodies are programmed to be able to survive just fine with regular breaks from eating. Not to mention how convenient it makes travel days, packed schedule days, and crazy meeting days.

What Caryn realizes is that you value your free time and don't want to spend it having to worry about the negative impact of work and travel. She also knows you can't wish excess weight away – you have to have a plan. I have used these tools and they absolutely work!!! If you take the time to apply them they will work for you, too. I wish you success in creating a life with enough time for all the things you want to do.

Angela L. Beauchaine, M.D., F.A.A.P.

Dedication

To Liv, for inspiring the journey, and to Todd for partnering in possibility.

Table of Contents

I Wanted It

These just might be the three most dangerous words in weight loss.

There are things I want all around me, all the time. I'm really good at wanting a Tesla and not having it. I wasn't as good at wanting a chocolate chip cookie and not having that.

Why is that? Habit. We're in the habit of seeing food, wanting it, and eating it. We say "I wanted it," believing that's enough justification. The desire for the cookie is normal, but our reaction to that desire is something we can choose.

That is what I needed to learn so that I could change my life. I needed to know that the cookie is less important than the life I am creating. I learned I can handle the short-term discomfort of not eating everything I want because I know where I'm headed and that long-term satisfaction is so much better than a cookie.

Is this book just about learning to say 'no' to a cookie? No, it's about building an awareness of your own food attitudes, and about cultural expectations around food. It's not about willpower; it's about changing your habits to support the person you want to be, the future you want to have.

Old habits will get you the same results you've been getting. If that isn't what you're after, then use the tools in this book to decide who your future – your ideal – self is. By following the steps I've outlined here, you won't need to wait for some future date to be your best self. You can put in the work and become her right now. Today.

Introduction

Conventional wisdom is keeping you fat. Yes, fat.

Six small meals a day keeps you fat.

Thinking you can eat a burger and run it off at the gym is keeping you fat.

Low-fat keeps you fat.

100-calorie snack packs are keeping you fat.

Eating breakfast to get your metabolism going is keeping you fat.

Eating overly processed "healthy" foods is keeping you fat.

What really gets me is that we all think we know what we should be doing to lose weight, but feel guilty that we aren't doing it. Your body is doing exactly what it's supposed to do - it's your big

human brain paired with conventional wisdom
that's getting in the way - and keeping you fat.
Yes. The *new* F word. It's uncomfortable even
typing it, but please stick with me.

*You're intelligent, successful in your career and
in so many other areas of life, and you can't help
but wonder, "Why am I still struggling with my
weight? Shouldn't I have this figured out by
now?"*

You work a crazy job that you're really good at
doing. People come to you because they know you
are someone who gets things done. You show up
in a big way for your work and for the people in
your life - no problem, no questions asked. Done.
You're smart, you're committed, and you take
care of business in every other area of life - but
weight loss remains elusive. Even with the best of
intentions - the right yoga pants, the protein
powder, all of it purchased and in place, the
weight never comes off. The "healthy lifestyle"
never fits or sticks.

You know that if you had three extra hours in the
day, or a second Sunday every week *then* you
could nail it. As it is, you have a mantra: You're

too busy to lose weight. You travel too much to grocery shop, let alone prep food or exercise enough. You're not in charge of your schedule. You *know* that if you just had a normal job where you stayed at home all the time you could finally lose weight and be healthy. Your work keeps you going constantly and there are crazy expectations of you and your time. You can't get away from that - nor do you want to.

You shouldn't have to choose between the life you've worked hard to create, and the body in which you want to live it.

You've tried the big name diets; you've read more books than you care to admit about how to lose weight. They've told you everything not to do, a few things to do, and a number of things that contradict each other. It's confusing out there but you're intelligent, you know what you need to do to lose weight -- IF you had the time to actually do it.

Every time you travel – which is a lot – your routines, all your progress, all your good intentions around eating go out the window. When you come home, it's often to a fridge full of not-much-good and a sink full of you're not sure what.

You're tired. You're busy. You do a lot. It's all true - and you want to be different.

You know that there are people out there who manage to pull this off, but you're pretty sure they don't have your job, your family, or your responsibilities. When life slows down, *then* you'll get started. You just need a little breathing room to make it happen. So you're going to take the weekend, catch your breath, unpack from the last two trips and start on Monday.

That mythical Monday never comes. Neither does January 1, nor the day after your birthday, nor the day after you get home from your much-needed vacation. Those fictitious start dates that hold the promise of the new world are just that – fictitious.

If you keep waiting, you will stay the same. You'll continue to be frustrated with the time you spend worrying about your weight. You'll never wear the skinny clothes you've been saving. You'll continue to be dissatisfied by spending money on clothes you don't like and in which you're not comfortable.

Or, you could show up.

Show up and be a grown up and learn again, not for the last time, that today is the only day you ever have - and even when it's hard and even when you are tired (because every day has some tired and some hard in it) - you show up so that you can pull the expensive jeans that you've only worn twice before out of the stack in the bottom corner of the closet, and wear them out of your house and into your life.

You show up so you can eat in a way that gets you the body you want. So you can eat out, and travel, and come home to normal life down a pound or two. You can get the body you want in the life you have. Yes, even you, with your job, and your busy schedule.

Imagine not caring about what food would be served at the meeting you are going to. Imagine knowing exactly what to order off any menu and knowing that you'll be satisfied every time. Imagine the possibilities if you had all the extra time you've been using to worry about your food and weight and you got to apply that to your life? Would that give you the extra hours you've been wishing you had?

Everything I do, everything I talk about in this book, is in service of that freedom. I see how hard you work to not care about food, to pretend indifference to something you really want. It's so exciting to imagine what you will do with all the extra brain space and time. I mean, if you really stop engaging with the struggle around food and your weight and live your life, what is possible?

You can be successful at this.

I know what you're thinking. You think you've been here before. You're reading another diet book, getting that all too familiar feeling of excitement about what will happen, how the weight is finally going to come off. Knowing the other shoe will drop, because that is what other shoes do... That could totally happen with this book too. It all depends on you and your knowing what you need to make it happen. Be willing to be onto yourself for this process. Be willing to drop the negotiations and be honest about why you're doing what you're doing and why you aren't doing what you you're not doing! That's it. Even if you don't do a damn thing other than read this chapter - be really clear about why you put the book down and aren't going to pick it back up.

I get that you've been lied to before and you've been shamed about your weight. You've been sold a story about how this works, and that story has set you up for failure. You've had your doctor tell you to lose weight while offering you next to no help, with a side of judgment.

You want this time to be different. You might even say you *need* this time to be different.

In the coming pages I share the groundwork for successful, sustainable weight loss, and tools for every trip, party, and event you will ever go to. Once you've got the plan, we'll address all the ways you are used to failing and what you can do to succeed this time.

I'm not talking about counting calories, worrying about what there is to eat on the plane, or putting your food in portion-sized containers. I've got you covered without the crazy diet baggage that has gotten you where you are today. You don't have to worry about where you're going to eat when your plane lands because you have a plan - a plan you can put into play anywhere.

You don't need to be special; you don't need to be "that person" with all their rules and special foods. You do need to show up, and keep showing up for yourself. Together we will streamline the weight-loss process in a way that is personal to you. We will end the daily struggle, and use skills you already have to get you the results you want.

It's time to make The Struggle as good as done.

Chapter 1: My Story

I'm a busy working mom and partner, I love my family and I don't spend enough time enjoying them. I travel for work and play often, and I value that part of my life. I am also a woman who has struggled, for the large majority of my life, with my weight. Or with my head about my weight, or my thoughts about how I should be different than I am. I didn't know how to do it though, and what trying to lose weight would mean for me, *about* me. Aren't I supposed to be okay with who I am? Even in this body, or the body I had - isn't it not feminist to care about this? But I do care!

I got what I should be doing or what I should look like - what I didn't get was how to lose weight and why I hadn't been able to. I thought about it a lot, it was really distracting. I was embarrassed to admit it, so I usually didn't - I kept my discomfort to myself. I took on and owned the role of Big Girl and that was great! I earned it; I was strong enough and athletic enough to pull it off for awhile. I did cool jobs that big strong girls do - commercial fishing, worked on boats, at a brewery - I just didn't want to make that okay anymore - and you don't have to.

As things began to click for me, I realized that the benefit was even bigger than I expected: Changing my approach to weight loss means that not only have I lost weight, I've also gained that time I used to spend engaged in The Struggle. The Struggle is all the should-haves, the I-knew-betters, the I'll-start-Mondays, the new diet books, the wishing, the regretting, the not wearing the bikini, the STRUGGLE. All the stuff we don't do because *weight*. All the stuff we do because *weight*. All the thoughts we think and bargains we make and time we spend hoping and counting and preparing and failing.

***Because weight*. It's the ultimate and inclusive excuse for ducking out of life**.

The Struggle will suck the life out of you and you won't be able to tell the difference between it and you. I was so entangled with The Struggle that I'm still picking out the rogue diet-y parts that pop up every once in awhile like lint in the corner of your jeans pocket. It's soft and seems normal so you don't even really know it's there and then BINGO! You get to that place where you're onto yourself again, and you take back your life a little bit more. You have that much more space, and it's freedom. THAT is why we're here - I'm here so that you can get free of The Struggle, find some more life and be a little more you a lot more often until one day you're not a dieter, you're not too big, you can tie your shoes easily, you don't fear the seat-belt extender. You're just you.

Where I Began

I paid $1200 to lose 20 pounds back in grad school. I was committed. I showed up. I ate the plan. I lost the weight. I wanted to puke during my workouts - it was bliss. Until it wasn't. I didn't have $1200 to drop on a trainer every semester along with my tuition. So I never saw him again - nor have I seen one since. I did keep the weight pretty much off, lost muscle, gained fat - stayed the same. I know you know the story - or a similar personalized version you paid to experience.

I thought I'd figured out what weight loss looked like, what it had to be:

13

You eat Special K cereal with soy milk and black coffee for breakfast, a yogurt and string cheese for snack, and lean beef with broccoli and grapes at dinner - oh and the same peppered turkey breast sandwich on wheat with mustard and greens - every day. Like magic. Forever.

You do cardio on your "off" days. You keep strength training next to those people who seem to live at the gym. You wish you felt comfortable trying a new class more often, you wish you were having a "these are my people" experience while sweating it out - but you're not.

Frustrated by this narrow view of weight loss and its accompanying sense of failure, I began to search farther afield. I had a big "Aha!" moment while reading the book <u>Intuitive Eating</u>. The clouds parted. THIS. THIS! It was like, "These ladies get it!" They are saying what felt so true, but nobody else was saying it.

You can trust your body. You can TRUST YOUR BODY! Wait what? Are they telling me my body knows better than all the experts to whom I'd rather outsource my weight problem?! <u>Intuitive</u>

<u>Eating </u>is a fantastic book about rebuilding body-image and making peace with food. Reading it changed my brain and welcomed my spirit. It was one of those books that put a crack in that boarded up, committed-to-the-struggle part of me that wasn't sure it was safe to hope.

So I intuitively ate. I ate what I wanted when I wanted. I tuned in to my cravings, I created more intimacy with my hunger, my body, my fullness. I stayed the same weight or within a 10-12 pound range for about 10 years. Not bad, right?! You might even say it was good, and for awhile it was! It felt good – I dressed well, I ate well — but I was still having thoughts that didn't feel that great. I was still obsessed with food. I still had the late night ice cream habit, I just didn't do it as often and I didn't beat myself up or throw myself off the wagon in the same way as I had in the past.

It was during this time of my life I became very aware of not being okay - and not being okay with not being okay. You know what I mean? Like, yeah, I eat healthy and I cook well but... I still eat all the cookies when no one is watching. I can stress eat my way through a bag of tortilla chips with the best of them. I still do all those things that I assume unhealthy people do - even if I'm eating organic! It was the habits and the patterns and the diet-like feelings that weren't working for me - no matter what the scale said. I knew there was more to this - I didn't know exactly what came next so I stayed the same for years. I stayed between the guardrails of what felt healthy and what felt too heavy.

Then I got pregnant. When I conceived I was at the very top of my weight fluctuation (two pounds heavier than when I worked with that trainer, but nowhere near as strong!). I had always told myself I'd be the healthiest I'd ever been when I got pregnant so the baby would have a great start (Read: so I would have the best chance at not gaining pregnancy weight that I would never lose.)

I kept it together during my pregnancy, I ate well, and not too much. I didn't gain weight very fast and it was mostly baby. Even pregnant, I only went up as high as my highest weight ever and that felt like an accomplishment. Then the same old thoughts and feelings came back. I might have done a great job of not getting fat while pregnant, but why? I still felt the same. I was still dissatisfied with how I felt and distracted by food. I still wanted to get the brownie with my

Starbucks latte at every airport.

I still wanted to overeat.

Making the Change

Though I didn't recognize it right away, something fundamental in me changed when I had a little girl. While pregnant, I'd found myself hoping for a boy, who might be more likely to be spared a lifetime of food issues. But the reality was that I was going to be raising a future woman and that she will be growing up in food and diet-obsessed, unhealthy and health-shaming America. I am excited to watch her grow up, to have a chance at saving her from some of the bullshit, but I also want to be realistic. She is a female, growing up in our world - can she be spared The Struggle?

Some people make it through unscathed, but I didn't. How do I do this without making it worse for her? How do I make it an issue without making it an issue? How do I create a space for her to be who she is in a body that feels comfortable for her?   How do I keep from imposing my struggle – The Struggle – on her?

I obviously had a lot of questions but I also had some fear. I was pissed I even had to even think about this! If I had a boy would it have been different? I don't know, but there I was - and I realized that if I didn't do this work right now then she may have to.

I got that if I didn't take care of my own stuff, clean up my brain, and get okay with whatever I am up to - she will know and she will feel it and I would regret that forever. I wanted - I *needed* - to be as onto myself about this as possible. I vowed that she would never see me sitting on a couch with a pillow on my lap to hide my body. She will see me in a swimsuit - swimming, laughing. She will see me being active in a body that feels like my own - that I feed well and move in ways that feel good *because* it feels good to me. Not because I am trying to punish it smaller.

A quote by Maya Angelou that I love is "When you know better you ought to do better." I knew that "better" existed, I knew I had the ability to create it - if I committed - and I wanted that for her and to do that I had to have it for *me* first.

Finding my Way

I value efficiency above most things - sometimes to my detriment. What that gave me in this situation is a strong urge to find the best way to lose weight and keep it off in the fastest way possible. I hired the best coach I know and I got to work. I did everything she said plus used what I already knew, kept at my own research, and made this crazy experiment my life.

I did it in service of myself and my daughter and all my clients to come. I had to know - what would work. Is thin possible? If it is - do I want it?

It is, and I do - and it's good enough that I want it for you too.

I stopped subscribing to popular culture and went my own way. Pioneering is not easy - and it's been everything. It's sort of like I've discovered a new land and this book is me sending word back to you about what is possible here. It's this crazy place where I can forget there is cake on a table. I weigh a new weight, one I don't even have a reference point for in adult life - and I don't even care because I am free. *Free.*

I know how to eat in any situation. I know how to fuel my body to get the results I want at home, on the road, on vacation - anywhere. I don't hide. I go out. I travel. I eat at restaurants. I cook. I am not afraid of food, or places, or eating with people. I want to live my life with food in it - not live my life around my food plan.

My Mission

I want to help other people because I am disgusted by the amount of time our culture spends obsessing about food. We have too many problems to solve, gifts to discover, books to write, people to become, to waste so much time on 100-calorie snack packs and other sad attempts at helping us lose weight.

Freedom. It's all, always, about freedom.

One of my clients is a working mom who travels constantly. She has almost no time for herself and had become very efficient at taking care of everything and everyone else, but she never made it onto her own to-do list. Her weight was evidence of how little she prioritized herself: She was 280 pounds when we started working together.

Things have changed. She signed up, did the work every day, came to our coaching calls, implemented everything we talked about, asked great questions, was thoughtful about her life and her choices, and has lost over 50 pounds. I have zero doubt that her weight loss will continue because she is committed - not to me or a number on a scale - but to herself. She is committed to creating a life that is sustainable and a body she wants to live life in. She uses the tools, works the plan - even when it's hard - and she shows up for herself.

You can do it too. Through this book you will build self-awareness, set concrete goals, develop a customized plan, and start becoming your best self. You will need to do the work, but the tools are all here. And if you need some extra help and support, I'm here too. Shoot me an email at caryn@caryngillen.com.

Caryn Gillen

Chapter 2: The Framework

You can lose weight AND travel. You can leave your house, eat at restaurants, go to people's homes, enjoy a picnic... You can live your life.

It is possible.

I want you to have access to the best information I know of to create the body you want so that you can live the life you want. When clients sign up for my coaching services, we work together to customize the structure of the process for their individual needs - which is ideal - but if it isn't in the cards for you right now I still want you to have the information you need to get the results you want!

I've maintained a 50-pound weight loss and helped my clients reach and maintain their goal weights, and I've learned that these tools work - when you use them. These tools are trustworthy and can be counted on. I get that the desire for this to not work will be strong because that's safer for you, and your brain wants to protect you from this big scary change. Make room for that possibility to exist. It doesn't mean you're in the wrong place, it just means you're normal. Managing your mind is an important part of the process - maybe the most important part.

I'm going to take you through my proven steps as if you're my client; it's your job to be onto yourself – tools for self-awareness and accountability are built into this program, but for them to work you have to be honest. Addressing our issues around food can be uncomfortable and unfamiliar, but it's an essential part of the process.

You can do this. I'm right here with you, let's do it together.

The tools in this book address the hardest part of weight loss: Your brain. I know, it sucks. I wish that I could hand you a vial of sparkly potion that you could spritz on your neck and then magically eat whatever you wanted whenever you wanted and weigh what you wanted... But since that doesn't exist, I'm going to help you tame and leave behind The Struggle so that you can live your life with all its ups and downs, trips, celebrations, daily cravings, AND still lose weight. So that your outsides match your insides and you can focus on living and creating this big beautiful life for yourself.

The Six Steps

Step One: **Prepare and Commit**

Step Two: **Build Awareness**

Step Three: **Recalibrate**

Step Four: **How to Eat**

Step Five: **Make Great Plans**

Step Six: **Putting it all Together: Travel with Ease**

I would love, love, love, to hear from you by email caryn@caryngillen.com or on my Facebook page (www.facebook.com/caryngillen) that you are killing it with your weight loss. Tag me in photos of you eating (or not) at the airport - whatever it is, stay in touch!

Let's do this.

Chapter 3: The Steps

Step One:

Prepare and Commit

This chapter is all about laying the foundation for a successful weight-loss journey. Through a series of worksheets you will set specific goals, identify what motivates you, and create a detailed vision of your very best future self.

Goal Weight

When I started losing weight, my goal was to weigh 175 pounds; it was my magic number. It wasn't always that far off from where I was - but it was a loooooong way. I imagine you have a magic number too, that elusive end goal you've had your mind on for awhile.

What's your number? Write it down.

Now subtract that number from your current weight. For example, if you weigh 200 and your goal is 175 your goal would be to lose 25 pounds. The healthy average pace of weight loss is six pounds per month. So, 25 pounds divided by 6 months is: 4.16 - we'll round up to 4.5. It's January first - you'll be at goal weight by Tax Day, April 15th. How does that sound? Sounds pretty good to me!

The problem is you can't do it using conventional wisdom - you can't restrict your calories all the way down to goal weight because that is not how the body works. I'm sure, in some way, you already know that. I'm sure you've tried calorie restriction in the past in hopes of weight loss and it probably worked at the start and then stopped working. That's because your body is so smart, it starts conserving energy in reaction to the lowered calories. It freaks out, thinks you're going to kill it. So it takes charge, slows your metabolism, and saves the day. It also leaves you at the same weight - or maybe even heavier than when you started.

In order for you to experience the six pound per month weight loss, you have to be willing do things differently: You have to challenge what you've been taught about how to lose weight. Use the steps in this book to work with your body to achieve the results you want.

Notice I said WITH your body. We're not doing this against your body - this is not a fight, it's a partnership. You don't need to feel overly hungry to lose weight, you don't need to eat rice cakes, you don't need to count calories, and you do need to eat fat. So please, please stick with me on this. Consider the reality that your body wants to feel great and live at a healthy weight too - but you have to be open to the process being collaborative. Your body is in. Are you?

Commit

If you want to lose weight, then you have to
commit. To yourself and to the process. This is
one of those things everybody says you have to do
but I did not get it until I signed up to work this
stuff out, to NAIL weight loss for the last time. To
end the generational food issues so that my
daughter doesn't have to have the struggle I've
had.

I'm not talking about a fuzzy kind of "Yeah! I'm
totally going to do that, just as soon as I do this
other thing first…" I'm talking about the kind of
committed where you know the minute you start
that you are as good as done. After completing my
own weight-loss journey, I now operate from goal
weight and future self, continuing the process of
becoming the woman I want to be in the world.
Whenever I decide to do anything - making jam,
writing this book, removing the wallpaper from
my entryway - it is as good as done. I know
beyond a shadow of a doubt that if I start, I finish.
So, I am very, very clear and purposeful when I
start things.

I want that for you because I know if you do that,
you will be successful. If you want to lose weight

and you want to be able to maintain or lose weight while you travel and live your busy, beautiful life you can have that. You can use all these tools to do that. How? You commit, and you keep committing. You show up for yourself. You be "onto yourself" about where you are slippery and where you will throw yourself under the bus, and where you need help and where you could get lost. Luckily, you know you better than anyone else so you're the perfect person for the job.

Identifying Your Key Motivator:

1. What is your goal weight?
2. How is that number going to change your life?
3. Why did you pick that number? Be really clear. What do you think it will give you?
4. What can you do at that number, in that body, that you can't do now?
5. What are you excited to do at that weight?
6. Who are you when you are at goal weight?
7. What does it feel like to be that person?
8. What are your primary feelings there?
9. Now hone in on those feelings and pick the top one.

That feeling is your **Key Motivator**.

Make a list of the 10 ways you can activate that feeling in your life now.

For example, my Key Motivator is "Grace."

I want to use that feeling, grace, to pull me forward into the life I'm creating. So, when I am feeling off my game or like I'm forcing something one way I tune back in is to ask myself "Is this graceful or grasp-y?" Asking that question almost instantly makes clear what my next step should be because I can feel into that future I am creating.

Today I spent some time self-coaching and checked in with that feeling of grace that comes so easily to my future self. Am I headed in the right direction? Is what I am creating feeling grace-filled? What is the goal I am trying to achieve and do my current plans and actions match up with that feeling in a way that makes sense and will help to keep me motivated?

Use your key motivator to propel you towards your goal weight and the life you are creating. Read or recite your ten beliefs so that you can conjure up that feeling as often as you can. You're practicing having the feeling you think is off in the future – and you're doing it now, in the present. You want to create time and space to manifest these positive feelings in your life now, at the weight you are now so that you can ride them all the way down to goal weight and be skilled at feeling them when you get there.

Create Your New Weight Beliefs

Often when we try and lose weight we punish ourselves into being different, without addressing our core beliefs about food, diet, and weight loss that have made – and kept - us overweight. It's time for you to change how you think, change your beliefs about losing weight, being thin, or – and this is key - who you are around food.

Here are some example thoughts from clients:

- ☐ I don't have time to lose weight.
- ☐ I travel too much; I can't plan meals like other people.
- ☐ I'd rather not lose that much weight, I just want to be healthy.
- ☐ I can't entertain clients without drinking.
- ☐ It's too hard to order at a restaurant.
- ☐ It's really hard to say no when I'm trying to rally the team or I'm hosting and I want everyone to be saying "Yes!"

Which of those have you thought before? What others can you add? Go ahead and write them down, take a minute to figure out what thoughts you have that are keeping you at the weight you're at right now. A trick to identifying these thoughts is that they may seem true - you probably believe them. So, question every belief you have and see if it's helping you or getting in your way.

Did you do it?

Good. Now you can see what you've been struggling against, maybe without even knowing. How does it feel to see that list? (If you have trouble with this exercise you are not alone - it is really hard to spot our own slippery beliefs! It can help to actually write them down.) What do you notice? Any themes?

Anything make you feel any particular feeling? Maybe that feeling is your key de-motivator? Watch out for it - it probably means you're thinking thoughts that are not going to get you the results you want!

Now that you've got a sense of the landscape, we are going to start fresh. We're not going to try and edit your beliefs because they are too old and well-worn.

We're going to create a brand new fresh set of beliefs. These new beliefs are going to get you the results you want - not the results you've had.

10 New Beliefs

A few examples of new thoughts are: "I have all the time I need to accomplish what I want to do." "I create the results I want for my body." "Eating while traveling is easier than eating at home."

1.
2.
3.
4.
5.
6.
7.
8.
9.
10.

Now that you've got them, use them. Read them every day. Read them aloud into your voice recorder on your phone and play them when you're in your car. Memorize them and allow yourself to feel the feelings that they evoke.

The three places and/or times of day I will recite my new thoughts are:

1.

2.

3.

Bonus: *Make sure you've got your Key Motivator coming through on at least three of these thoughts.*

Write The Future

I will talk a lot in this book about your future self, about how this is a journey of not only weight loss, but also self-awareness. The choices you make today are in service of the person you want to become, the person you are becoming. This exercise will help you define just who your future self is.

Take ten minutes and sit down with some paper or a journal. You can pick the month you expect to end up at goal weight, or I like to pick today's date one year from now and write as if it is that day and all the changes I've been working on are made. The person you have been creating is the person writing.

Let her say whatever she wants. She may get you updated on some of the smaller details of life but as she does I want you to notice who she is. Can you get a sense of her primary emotions? What is she focused on, what is the next step for her?

Make sure you have her spend some time reflecting on what she did that was so helpful in getting her where she is; she has much wisdom to share with you.

Caryn Gillen

Step Two:
Build Awareness

Awareness is to permanent weight loss as gluten is to bread: It's what holds it together and makes it resilient. The person who has your desired result - the result you committed to when you identified your Key Motivator, created your new beliefs, and who helped you write the future – they use the three tools in this chapter every day.

Weigh Every Day

Yes, every damn day. I know! You would so rather *not* do that for all sorts of good reasons, I'm sure! My client Gerri thought once per week was more "reasonable" and that it was more fun to see the number go down in bigger increments. I get it - and I still want you to do it every day.

I want you to do this is so that you start seeing that number as a data point. You're checking in, creating awareness. I don't want to hear from you that you got on the scale and gained ten pounds without even noticing. Checking in and gathering data is helpful so that you can stay accountable to yourself. It may seem like it's easier to overeat, check out, and not think about the food or the meal planning - but the truth is we are never *not* thinking about it! You're spending your brain space and energy on The Struggle anyway. Keeping track of your weight – without judgment or fear – is a way to let go of that.

Another reason weighing yourself every day is helpful is that you start to know your body better. We have hormones doing things we don't always notice, taking care of us without our knowledge. My client Amy has a 26-day weight-loss cycle. She doesn't lose weight until days 20-26. She has to hold on for 20 days without the number on the scale moving. Had she not kept a food journal (more on that in a moment), and tracked her weight every day, she wouldn't have known that and those 20 days would have remained excruciating. It's hard to give effort and not see the results you want to see, but if you knew that the results were coming – that they were a sure thing - wouldn't you stick with it?

I weighed myself all the way down to goal weight - and then down three more pounds from there and I still weigh every day. One interesting thing I learned is that I had always associated being thin or not weighing very much with being "weak." Some days at 142 I did feel really weak and I would think "See, this isn't sustainable, I knew it!" Then other days I felt amazing, strong, clear and confident in my body and when I got on the scale and it said 142 it surprised me. That highlighted and challenged my belief that thin = weak. So, the numbers can be deceptive. That doesn't mean we don't use them as a tool, it just means how you feel is also a tool. When I feel weak at 142 I can discover it's because I have been eating well but not as quality as usual and I've probably spent too much time sitting at my desk and skipped yoga for a week or two. How you feel in your body is more important than what the scale says, but what the scale says is still useful.

I want that kind of awareness for you, too. I want you to be surprised and proud of what your body can do, and to be responsive to what you know it needs based on how you feel in your skin - not because anyone tells you to but because you've created this intimate relationship with yourself and you know better than anyone else what you need. It's important to remember that there is no thought we can't use to increase our awareness about our relationship with ourselves, and to help us be successful in our weight loss.

Hunger Scale

McKenzie was always in a hurry to eat by 7 pm, which had nothing to do with her hunger and everything to do with a food rule her mom had at their house. Her mom believed – and built the family's food schedule – around the idea that to be "healthy" (to stay trim), people shouldn't eat after 7 pm. That idea stuck with McKenzie, but it didn't work for her. She was rushing to eat by 7 pm, but it wasn't getting her the results she wanted. As of today, she's has lost 30 pounds, which can be at least in part attributed to her letting go of an old food rule and tuning into her own body's signals.

Using the Hunger Scale helps you tune into your body and your hunger by discovering *why* we do what we do, and challenging old food, diet, or "healthy lifestyle" rules we may be holding on to that aren't helping us. If we're not hungry and we go for a snack, it's pretty clear we are eating for entertainment or some reason other than hunger.

Below you'll find the Hunger Scale worksheet with some descriptions to help you get an idea of how to label your hunger, but you'll need to define

47

them for your own body. A +4 for you might feel different than a +4 for me. I'd take some notes on what you feel in your body at certain points to get to know this better. Often times, there's only a bite or two between each of the numbers.

My client Cathy keeps a printed version of the Hunger Scale on her fridge, another client keeps it in her purse, and yet another on her phone. Whatever method works best for you, keeping this tool handy will increase its effectiveness!

Every time you eat anything you'll want to assign a number to your hunger/fullness level at the time you start and at the time you stop eating.

See the scale below as an example to get your started:

Hunger Scale

10 - You just had the biggest Thanksgiving meal of your life, you wish it was tomorrow so you could be done with this gross feeling.

9, 8, 7...

6 - Uncomfortably full, not energetic, you want to put your feet up.

5 -

4 - Stomach full, you don't need more food, not uncomfortable.

3 -

2 - You could eat more, or go for a walk, not lethargic.

1 -

0 - Neutral, absence of hunger, absence of fullness.

-1 -

-2 - A few hunger pangs. You could wait to eat and be okay.

-3 -

-4 - Hungry for awhile, starting to distract you.

-5 -

-6 - You're 'starving.'

-7, -8, -9...

-10 - You're so hungry you'd eat anything.

The Food Journal

People who keep a Food Journal – and keep it faithfully – lose weight the fastest and most consistently.

Even though I have been at my goal weight for a long time, I still keep a Food Journal every day. I know it's what made me lose weight so fast, keep it off, and gives me the confidence that the weight will remain off. When my clients aren't submitting their journals, chances are they're not losing weight.

I know you'll be too busy. Too much will be going on to get your Food Journal done. You'll want to wait until after that upcoming ___to really get started. I want you to challenge yourself here. Expect it to be uncomfortable to start this new habit - and then do it anyway. It's uncomfortable to lose weight - you have to do things differently than you've done before, and changing the norm doesn't feel normal! Please consider that it will take you fewer than five minutes to do this each day.

Is making the change you want to make -

the goal you identified at the start of this book, the healthier lifestyle, the coming home lighter from trips - is that worth five or fewer minutes of being thoughtful with yourself each day?

If it isn't - if you don't want to do this, that's totally fine. We're cool - just stop reading, pass this book on to a friend, and get on with your life. If you choose this option, own that! It is fine to be who you are today - as long as it is working for you and you are okay with the results. If you're not sure of your decision, not sure about the five minutes, just do the Food Journal anyway and we'll see what happens. Trust yourself that much, be willing to at least experiment with the idea of being "onto yourself." This process is about much more than you writing down your food each day, it's about increasing self-awareness, being accountable, and taking good care of *you*.

There are a number of ways you can keep your Food Journal: Note apps on your smartphone, Google Docs, Evernote, a paper notebook. Whatever you choose, be sure you keep up with yourself. If there is a change you could make to make it easier - do that right away. The process is much more important than the method even if it's a Post-It in your back pocket, you're doing it right. You'll want to get confused about how to do it or what to use to track it - don't fall prey to your confusion - it's just your brain resisting change.

How to Keep a Food Journal

Write down everything that goes in your mouth. Every bite, sip, taste. Yes, even when you taste the batter! Yes, even that one sip of your friend's drink. Just do it. Everything, every time.

Write:

- [ ] The time you ate.
- [ ] Where you were on the Hunger Scale when you started eating and where you were when you stopped. (See example below)
- [ ] Jot down any extra thoughts or notes about situations, especially if they led to overeating. Be your own best accountability partner.
- [ ] Weigh yourself at the same time each day and write that down too. If you notice that a thought comes up while you are on the scale, put that in your journal as well.

Food Journal example:

7-9 am 2 cups coffee with heavy cream -2 to 1.

No scale in hotel. I feel pretty much the same as the last few days though, I bet I'm the same or maybe down one pound.

Everyone was having pancakes but I hadn't planned them for my Joy Eat so I focused on connecting with people over breakfast instead of thinking about missing out on food.

Noon: -4 to 4. Taco salad with everything - had them serve it in a bowl instead of the big shell. Iced tea.

3:30 - They brought out cookies - I didn't know they'd have those, I totally wanted one - they distracted me for about 10 minutes until I thought "I didn't plan them today but if I really want I can have a cookie tomorrow." I know I won't plan it but that sure felt better than the thought

"I can't have it!"

6:30 As planned, I did happy hour with my team. I specifically looked ahead at the menu and found the items I wanted to order for everyone so I knew I'd have things I wanted to eat with them. I had said I could have 3 drinks, I had two, it was enough. I do notice I get really distracted from my hunger/fullness levels when I drink, so I'm not sure what the numbers were. I wasn't hungry when I got back to my room - I did want to snack but I didn't.

It's important to record the details. These can help you see patterns, notice challenges, and it builds awareness around your food habits. You may notice you always overeat when you hang with certain friends. You may notice your weight goes up the day after you eat red meat, or that you don't lose weight when you don't drink enough water. The Food Journal is not a place for judgment; it isn't where you go to feel bad about what you've done. It's a helpful, sometimes boring investigation into the choices you make, why you're making them, and what happens when you do.

My clients share their Food Journals with me every day. It allows me to see everything in real time so we can start to identify patterns and potential pitfalls, and also so we can celebrate successes. Do the same for yourself. Show up and tell the truth for yourself. If you don't like what you are writing down or the results you're creating, then use that as motivation to stick to the program and make some changes that you're proud of - not because of what the scale says, but because you're honoring your commitments to yourself.

Step Three:

Recalibrate

In this chapter we start to make adjustments to your diet that will kick-start the weight loss process and change your relationship to your body's fuel.

Reset Your Hunger

If you feel like your hunger is urgent or constant, if you feel like you've messed up your metabolism with crazy diets and overeating, or just feel like you're not on the right track, then it's time to recalibrate. Recalibration will get you into a position where you can feel normal hunger and fullness cues. The best way I know how to do that is to remove flour and sugar from your diet. I know that you don't want to hear that because I didn't want to hear it either! I'm saying it anyway.

Taking the white powders out of the equation means creating trustworthy lines of communication between your body and your brain. This will help you to increase fat burning (weight loss) and that's what we're going for, right? We want your body to learn how to use the fat it already has on board for fuel. I know we've all had the thought "Why am I hungry? Why can't my body just tap into this fat that's hanging all over me so I can lose some weight?" It can, but not until you teach it how to use fat for fuel. The problem is that your body is used to the easy solution, it would rather burn carbohydrates than fat stores for fuel because it's easier - and it's what it is used to do.

I'm pretty sure that at this point you want to stop reading and maybe throw this book away and you may have even said "Yeah, whatever lady!" in your head.

Personally, I was scared. I wasn't sure I *could* do it. I wasn't sure I could last more than an afternoon. I remembered a time I'd gone on a crazy cleanse where all I ate was chicken and vegetables and eggs and I had insane headaches and felt nauseous all day long - before going to bed at 8 pm so I could just escape the pain and suffering. This isn't that, but if you're afraid I get it, and I've been there, and I have to tell you that this time was different. I wasn't doing this as a fad cleanse - I was changing my life, my world, my family, and my future. Imagine what a badass you'll feel like when you truly don't crave sugar - like - you don't even care about it. It's pretty empowering! So no, it won't be easy and it may hurt a little in the beginning, but it will change everything. Depending on what your body is used to processing for fuel now will determine how much you will feel the adjustment as you switch over to no sugar and no flour.

I know it's a big deal, but a big deal with big results.

Your brain and body respond to concentrated, processed foods in the same way they respond to drugs. Eating a tablespoon of corn sugar is very different from a tablespoon of corn. Think about an orange. It's great when eaten as a part of your meal but orange juice is another ballgame as far as how your body reacts. You'd never sit down to eat the number of oranges it takes to make that glass of juice - you'd be too full from the fiber and bored with all the peeling. When foods are taken from their whole and natural state, they give fast, big, instant energy hits that your brain sees as rewarding and your body sees as easy fuel. Both brain and body say "Give me more of that!" Hello cravings - and the cycle perpetuates itself.

When I completely remove flour and sugar from my diet I like my brain better and I like my body better, which means I like my life better. That is the point of all of this. So if I said I can give you this tool and it will make everything better - would you do it? I hope you at least try it!

No Flour

No flour means no flours. No grains that were once whole that are now powder. Not ground up rice flour instead of whole wheat. Not gluten free - we aren't talking gluten, we're talking flours.

No Sugar

No sugar means no caloric sweeteners. Honey, agave, cane sugar, high fructose corn syrup, brown rice syrup, maple syrup - none of them. Not even if they're organic! You're welcome to experiment with calorie free sweeteners but the goal isn't to figure out how to eat a bunch of sweet food that you can handle and get away with, the goal is to tune your body into being able to crave real whole foods that serve it well.

Fat Adaptation

Giving up flour and sugar is the first step in making your body fat-adapted. Fat adaptation simply means your body relies on burning fat for fuel rather than using carbohydrate, or sugars. To become fat-adapted, you have to get to the point where you are relying on fat for your fuel and your body has stopped the need/craving cycle for carbohydrate.

The more excess fat you have on your body, the more you have to burn and the more you'll want to be aware of how you're using your meals to optimize the fat-burning times. Things can get a little rough for people when they are in fat-burning mode and are using a lot of the fat on their bodies for fuel. You could be burning fat that was stored weeks, years, or even decades ago - that just doesn't feel as good as burning a Caesar salad you ate tonight - but it works, and it's what you're going for. It's been called "burning dirty." I know some clients like the feeling because they know it's an indicator that their body is burning their fat for fuel and that their efforts are paying off. That said, not everyone feels it in that way. Your response to burning your own fat for fuel may be different, you may feel just fine.

You'll have to feel out, for your body, what works for becoming and staying fat-adapted. For example, how much complex carbohydrate (beans, rice, squash...) can you eat and not have your body resort to the more urgent carbohydrate-fueled kind of hunger? How much fruit works for you to still get the goals you want? Do you need protein every day, or maybe you find that chicken doesn't sit well but you have to have beef at least once a week. You'll want to eat fat at every meal and get a large portion of your fuel from fat. In the next chapter I'll talk in detail about the process of becoming fat-adapted, and share specific foods and menus that support not only optimal fat burning, but freedom from cravings and unmanageable hunger.

Caryn Gillen

Step Four:

How to Eat

In Step Three you did the work of eliminating two major players that get in the way of you having clear lines of communication with your body: Sugar and flour. You're probably already noticing that things are calmer, that maybe your hunger isn't as frequent or urgent, or that your sweet tooth is no longer as intense. As the dust continues to settle it's time to start the next step of this process: Tuning in. Part of this is about how you eat and the other part is about how you "be." Both are equally important to unlocking the path to your lighter self.

Meals Not Snacks

Eat meals, not snacks. Your body needs to have opportunities, when it's not processing food, to burn the fat you already have on board. So it can lose weight, a little bit every day until you hit goal weight - and then maintain it for the rest of your life. Make your meals big and satisfying. The kind that stretch your stomach out so you get the benefit of the hormone Leptin being secreted and telling your brain you are satisfied. The best way to do this is to have lots of veggies to increase the volume of the meal. You'll also want to be sure to have plenty of fat to satiate you and keep you satisfied between meals. When you are done with your meal, stop eating, and don't eat again until your next big satisfying meal. This idea of big meals instead of small meals or snacking throughout the day goes against a lot of what we've been told and sold for years. You may be feeling skeptical and I did too – until I tried it and it worked, not just for me, but for my clients too.

You may feel hunger between meals, this is normal and not an emergency (I know, this was news to me!) Here's the best part: Once you are fat-adapted, you'll experience hunger in a different way. It's gentler and easier to coexist with - the urgency is gone. Real physical hunger comes in waves and doesn't require an immediate response. When my client Maggie and I first started working together, she referred to it as the "Dangerous Hunger." After just a couple months of coaching, Maggie easily eats on protocol (more on that in a minute) and is no longer living in fear of her own hunger. Using the Hunger Scale from Step Two will help you start to recognize the difference between cravings and hunger.

Take my client Lisa, after beginning to work with me, she lost 20 pounds relatively quickly and was totally weirded out by her lack of hunger. She would write things in her Food Journal like, "How could it be that I could go until 3 pm and really not want to eat lunch? So I ate the salad I brought because I know I'll have to eat dinner at 6 with the family." I love hearing things like this from my clients for two reasons: One they are fat-adapted and have freedom from that gnawing hunger that has ruled so many of our lives and minds, and two, it's more proof that we have been encouraged to not listen to or trust our bodies to tell us what they need (and we can change that!).

So the next question you ask is: Do you have to

eat when you are not hungry?

No. I know it seems like an obvious answer, but the next time it's noon and everyone is eating and you aren't hungry - try it. Habit and culture are hard to challenge - no matter what your goals are. Not being hungry when you are trying to lose weight is perplexing, different, and it takes some getting used to. The next step for Lisa was to not eat when she wasn't hungry; to honor her body and do what she needed to do to get the results she wants. That can look like dealing with a husband who's annoyed that she's not eating when everyone else is eating, or it could be her willing to feel sad that she doesn't get to eat with everyone at work - and addressing that emotion with something other than food. It may be easier for her in the moment to just eat - and that is what she would have done in the past and it's likely one of the reasons she's overweight. The challenge now is to do life where all the same challenging things come up - but do it differently. She needs to be connected to what she is creating (goal weight) so that it's easier to sit in the short-term discomfort knowing she's creating that long-term reward.

A big motivator for me, and something that made

it easier to sit with my hunger, was learning the science behind insulin and how it relates and can support weight loss. When you eat a snack, a meal, or even just a quick bite, your body has an insulin response. Some foods make it spike higher than others, in general you can think about it as sugar or simple carbohydrates (Juice, candy, baked goods...) getting the biggest rise and fat (Nuts, cheese, avocados...) getting the lowest. This is important because your body is in one of two modes: it's either processing the food you ate and working to get the insulin level down (burning or storing glucose) or it's working to turn your fat into energy it can burn. If you want to lose weight you want it to be in that mode as often as possible.

Meals not snacks support that science. You want to avoid quick bites here or there, or those handfuls of insulin spiking foods, or quick tastes during meal prep. You want to eat meals, like I describe above, that don't contain all the simple carbohydrates that make your insulin levels rise and cause your body to have to work long and hard to get those levels down. If you must snack, choosing something that doesn't cause your insulin level to spike will help you get back into fat burning mode the fastest.

These higher fat, bigger volume meals will work differently than you're used to. If you've been running primarily on carbohydrates for fuel you'll be happily surprised.

Establishing Your Protocol

Your protocol is simply the food you eat consistently that gives you the results you want - or not. For example, if you wanted to stay the same weight you are today you could look back at what you typically eat, create a list of the foods that you consume on a regular basis and keep eating that same way. That would be your current protocol. If you look back and notice that there is a pattern that's not working for you, you can change it up. The main point here is that you spend less of your time thinking about food and more time living and enjoying your life outside of eating.

When I started this journey I had a pretty regular protocol of foods that kept me overweight. I would eat two eggs with a tortilla, greens, and cheese each morning. I always wanted and usually had pizza on Sunday nights and nachos on Friday nights. I often ate leftovers for lunch and typically something sweet every day. Usually my husband and I had a curry or stir-fry one night a week and would eat leftovers from that for a few days. We were doing okay, we ate a lot of vegetables, we bought organic, and we cooked at home most of the time. The problem for me was that sugar was such a motivator, I would go out of my way to get it and get it often. I was also hungry (*hangry*) a lot. My husband would pack granola bars for me because I wasn't always the kindest hungry person!

My protocol now is to eat a lot of vegetables and a lot of satisfying fat. I usually start my day with some form of bulletproof or fatty coffee. There are lots of different recipes for this, most use a combination of grass-fed butter, coconut oil, medium chain triglyceride (MCT) oil, or heavy whipping cream. I use about 1.5 cups of coffee with a tablespoon each of grass-fed butter and coconut oil. I've used MCT oil and that worked well too, but I prefer the taste of coconut oil and I always have it around so it's easy. I'd love to use heavy whipping cream because that'd be even easier - but that much un-aged dairy doesn't work well for my body.

Then I eat a big salad for lunch. I build my salads upside down when I take them to the office so whatever greens I'm using don't wilt. I'll have seeds, cheese, ground flax, sour cream or yogurt and salsa as dressing, cooked and raw veggies and romaine and spinach on top. Sometimes I'll do a burger salad where the dressing is mayo and mustard. Basically it's a lot of veggies that are used as a vessel for the fat (cheese, dressing, avocado, egg, bacon...).

Dinner has a bit more variety than lunch but is often a salad as well. I think it's important to note that the addition of fat to your meal is more important than protein. You want to be sure you're getting the majority of your calories from fat.

You don't need to count calories but you do need to pay attention to what is working and creating the results you want for your body.

I know for me that if I start eating too little fat I'll start craving carbohydrates. The answer isn't to eat more carbohydrates, that's just my body telling me it wants fuel and what it needs is fat. When I've been doing really well at eating fats and veggies but it's been a number of days since I've had a complex carbohydrate (bean, squash, rice, potato, lentil...) my energy starts to go way down and I feel a bit depleted. I'm aware that this can happen, so I make a point to eat a complex carbohydrate every couple of days, every 4th day at the most. This is what feels right for me, what feels right for your body may be different. I've included a food list at the end of this section to give you some ideas, and here's a quick reference of how to eat a fat-adapted diet:

1. If you have a sugar craving, eat fat.
2. If you are going to eat an apple or some other fruit be sure and eat cheese or nuts or another kind of fat (bacon wrapped anything anyone?!) with it so that you're reducing the spike of insulin.
3. If you are struggling with how to eat this much fat after being encouraged for so long to eat a low-fat diet, consider starting with the "healthy" fats: Coconut oil, avocado, nuts, nut butters, eggs... You can absolutely do this without eating bacon and cream at every meal.
4. If you like lattes or mochas skip the low-fat/no-fat dairy. When they remove the fat it makes the overall sugar content of the dairy go up. Try ordering a latte with ⅓ heavy whipping cream, ⅔ hot water. It tastes more creamy than a regular latte, has more satisfying fat, and is less total sugar than a breve (a latte made with ½

and ½). For the mocha, do the same thing and add sugar free chocolate.

5. Skip low-fat dairy all together! Eat whole fat yogurts and sour creams.

6. If you're searching for recipes use the terms "High fat low carb" or "HFLC Recipes."

7. Peanut butter is fantastic – just make sure you're using the kind without all the sugar in it! All you should see on the ingredients list is "Peanuts and Salt." I stir mine with a bread hook attachment on my hand mixer and then refrigerate it so it doesn't keep separating.

Your Food Journal is an invaluable tool for figuring out what works best for your body. If, after working through the first four steps of this program, you still find yourself eating in the absence of physical hunger, shoot me an email and we'll see what's up: caryn@caryngillen.com .

Below is a list of some of the foods you could eat, it isn't a complete list by any means and it also isn't a must eat list. There are things here that may not work well for your body but work great for someone else. Like with every offering in this book, experiment, feel it out, and be willing to change it up in service of your goals.

Food List

Fats
Coconut oil, grass-fed butter, olive oil, butter, nut butters, olives, avocados, heavy whipping cream, eggs, bacon, mayonnaise, sour cream, flax seed oil, sesame oil, full-fat dressings, ghee, nuts, lard.

Vegetables
Asparagus, broccoli, carrots, tomatoes, green beans, bok choy, chard, kale, onion, peppers, radish, cauliflower, leeks, snap peas, celery, lettuce, beets, parsnip, okra, sprouts, radicchio, corn, spinach, squash, zucchini, yam.

Protein
Eggs, fish, beef, pork, chicken, shellfish, tofu, tempeh, lentils, seeds, nuts, cheese, yogurt, beans.

Grains
Rice, quinoa, oats, corn tortillas, grits, oat bran.

Fruit
Apples, banana, grapefruit, pear, orange, berries, peach, nectarine, plum, kiwi, apricot, pineapple, figs, mango, cherries, melon.

Caryn Gillen

Step Five:

Make Great Plans

In this section I'll set your mind at ease. Don't worry - you don't have to give up cake forever! You just have to plan for it - and introduce important tools that allow you to plan for any event.

We only have so much willpower to use each day. You can use it on decisions about what to eat, or you can use it on the things in life that you care about more than food and eating. Choosing to make decisions ahead of time about your food means you don't have to decide in the moment to be "good" or "bad" - you just do what you said you'd do, or you don't and you deal with the consequences of that (brain chatter, weight gain, getting better at cheating on yourself). We all think that we don't have enough time to plan our food and I get it, we're busy. I don't know about you, but I'm also kind of over using that as an excuse. Who's NOT busy?! There are people who do this, so why *not* you? Who would you have to be to make this a priority?

One thing I like to do for my clients is time how long it takes them to plan their eating for tomorrow while we're on the phone today. Here's what's really crazy: It's usually twenty-nine seconds or less. *Twenty-nine* seconds or less between you and weight loss. I'm not kidding. Twenty-nine seconds you guys, come on!

So now that we've blown "too busy" out of the water, there are other reasons why we don't want to plan and my client Katie is a great example. She's a foodie and was sure that she couldn't make this work because - she's a foodie! She felt like she needed to be able to cook whatever she wanted whenever, and make spur-of-the-moment decisions about what to eat. That is all totally fine, except that doing that wasn't getting her the results she wanted.

I was so happy when she voiced her objection to planning, because then we could address the beliefs that support that objection. After some discussion, we found out that for her, being a "foodie" means that she sources local foods, eats grass-fed meat, buys organic, and cooks interesting, delicious things with good flavor and spice. Once we had this clearly defined, it was obvious that the barrier to planning wasn't her being a foodie, it was her brain. Her brain was telling her that being a foodie meant it was impossible to plan. Once she realized that she didn't have to stop being a foodie to lose weight, she was happy to spend her 29 seconds a day to make food plans!

You have to be onto yourself. You have to be aware that your thoughts about planning, about giving up sugar, about anything, are just sentences in your brain - they are not necessarily the truth! Believing your thoughts is a choice. Allowing yourself to be confused is a choice. Change is a choice. You have to be willing to challenge yourself to change yourself. That's how you know you're doing it right.

Planning your meals doesn't mean deprivation – it just means deciding ahead of time when you'll have your treats. It doesn't mean you skip the party, or spend a trip sequestered in your hotel room to avoid temptation. This chapter contains three tools to help you think ahead (and reduce the need for willpower in the heat of the moment): Joy Eats, Event Plan, and Exception Plans.

Joy Eats

I see Joy Eats as the thing that makes eating this way human and sustainable. They mean you get to do what you want – as long as you plan for it. It's a practice, and just like you are practicing eating food for fuel the rest of the time, Joy Eats are the practice of eating purely for entertainment, for enjoyment. One time every week you eat something that is off protocol, just for the pleasure of it.

A lot of people wonder why they would do this if they are trying to lose weight. Losing sight of your goals often happens when you feel restricted, and if you feel restricted for long enough you want to bust free, eat a whole bag of kettle corn and say "F*ck it!" We've been taught to feel guilty about eating pleasurable foods. This practice of Joy Eating will challenge that and challenge you to plan ahead so that you can eat foods that have been vilified, or that contain flour and sugar, out in the open with a clean conscience.

Joy Eats happen once per week, every week. You want to get good at feeling the feelings that a Joy Eat can bring up. You might get excited for it, wait for it all week long, try to avoid it - it's all useful information. Whatever happens, they are planned at least one day in advance so that you're not reacting to or having to manage your lizard brain in the moment.

Whenever I see a cupcake of course my brain goes "I want that." The point of planning in advance is to outsource your decision making to your smarter human brain, to the person you are when you are making good plans. Have you ever decided on Sunday that at 3 pm on Monday you'll drop everything you're doing and eat 1/2 of a stale donut from the conference room? No, I haven't either - but I've sure eaten that stale donut. Now if I want a donut, I go to the best donut shop in town and I get the exact donut I want when I know it is fresh and I sit down with a hot cup of really good coffee and I enjoy it and move on with my day - no guilt. That's the difference between reacting and planning. That's a Joy Eat.

When Joy Eating, you want the Haagen-dazs not the Skinny Cow! It can be a meal or a dessert - but not both. The point of a Joy Eat is not to get to binge and 'narc out' on food for a day or an evening - the point is to consciously enjoy something that you like and isn't on your protocol. I look forward to my Joy Eats. I often do them at home where I can savor something instead of out where I am distracted By people, toddlers, busy places, etc. That works for me - you'll find out what works for you as you practice it.

Another aspect of the Joy Eat is you get to do it and move on. No guilt, no second guessing. You chose it, planned it, did what you said you'd do. Maybe it didn't feel how you thought it would - that's okay. They're not random or unplanned - they don't happen to you - you create the experience of them and sometimes it won't meet your expectations. This is normal.

This is not how you plan your Joy Eat: "Well, I haven't had my Joy Eat this week, so I'll just have this burrito that my co-worker brought in." That is *not* a Joy Eat - that's just being sloppy with yourself. Burritos are fine - I don't want you to miss the point here - it is the planning and following through that we are working on. When you see something you want - note that desire. Is that what you want for your Joy Eat this week? If it is, can you come back and get it when you have planned it?   Can you take some home for tomorrow?

When you see something you want and think, "I can't have that," it leads to feeling deprived. In this case, you can have that. You can have whatever you want. Plan your Joy Eats ahead of time, look forward to them, and en*joy* them!

Event Plan

This tool will help you prepare for any event – family gatherings, social dinners, holiday parties - by making your decisions ahead of time about your food, and addressing any challenges you may face. This plan allows you to see potential obstacles ahead of time and plan for them so that you have the best chance at enjoying the trip, party, or event.

You'll want to set aside some time to focus so you can be thoughtful with your answers. Be as detailed as you can!

1. What is the event?
2. What will be challenging about it?
3. What do you want to do? What is your plan? Your commitment?
4. What is your specific plan to carry this out?
5. When you get to the event how will you try to justify or excuse not following this plan?
6. Visualize three scenarios where you are challenged and you take the action you want to take.
7. If it gets really hard what is your plan?
8. Write a mantra that you could say quietly in your head.

Example:

1. What is the event?
   The event is a date with a friend at a favorite cheese shop and bar.

2. What will be challenging about it?
   I will want to over drink and then overeat because that is what I do with this friend and with wine and cheese!

3. What do you want to do? What is your plan? Your commitment?
   I want to drink 1-3 glasses of wine and eat delicious cheese and meats and olives. My decision ahead is to also drink water, eat and drink with her like usual but not get drunk and not over drink as an excuse to jump off the wagon and eat all the baguette in sight and

grab a cupcake on my way home. My commitment is to myself the next morning who has to be productive, who gets a morning to herself to drink coffee and write. I want to break this habit because

I love my mornings - my 'me' time and I don't want to throw away my mornings so that I can have food that hurts me or another glass of wine that WILL leave me hung-over.

4. What is your specific plan to carry this out?
My specific plan is to order sparkling water the moment we sit down, the big bottle. Then look at the whole menu, actually I'll look at the menu ahead so I have an idea and can just spend my time visiting with her rather than staring at a menu. So, I'll know exactly what I want. She doesn't eat

meat so I'll just pick one meat to order for myself. Any kind of veggies would be good too or a side salad. I am going to drink red wine and I'll pick my 3 glass options or a few bottle options if we go that route. I'll also pick out the kind of tea/coffee I want to order if I'm having any trouble at all stopping with the wine! The sparkling water will continue throughout the night.

5. When you get to the event how will you try to justify or excuse not following this plan?

   a. We're never out, what will it hurt?

   b. I'll just have a bite (when she orders dessert).

   c. I wish I could have that (I made my plan, I could have had that! Stick to the plan.)

   d. I never do things like this, it's okay.

e. *I don't want to be someone who goes out and limits herself.*

6. Visualize three scenarios where you are challenged and you take the action you want to take.

a. *She'll want to order a second bottle. I know if we order it, I'll drink it. I have my 3 glass choices already chosen so I will suggest that I just want a glass of_.*

b. *She'll ask if I want to order dessert. I will want to - I can expect that! I will say "That sounds amazing but I'm not feeling it tonight." Then I'll get right back to enjoying her company - which is why I'm there in the first place.*

c. *There will be delicious looking bread served with our cheese* and meat, I'll want to eat it at some point, probably after one glass of wine (it makes sticking to the plan harder!). I will know that that is coming and remind myself "Look at that! Right on time, I always want the bread but I still don't eat it. I'm awesome at this game."

7. If it gets really hard: My plan is to sit back, put my glass down and just breathe in the space. Enjoy the decor and the ambiance, we love this spot. I love my friend, I love hearing about her life. I love that I have someone I care about who I actually want to share and connect with. Breathe all that in and remember how much of it has nothing to do with the food or the beverages.

8. Write a mantra that you could say quietly in your head.

Mantra: *"Spending one-on-one time with people I love is my most favorite thing."*

Exception plan

This tool is for any time you want to go off protocol. It isn't a Joy Eat, it isn't an event - but you are going to eat off protocol. What that means is you are signing up for planned buffering from your life. Using this tool you will get clear on the consequences so you don't have to feel bad later.

1. Date
2. Why I'm making an exception
3. Action Plan
4. Consequences I am signing up for

Example:

1. Date
   September 25 - my brother's birthday.

2. Why I'm making an exception
   My sister-in-law is cooking ribs and there is bbq sauce on them - and I love them. I don't ever eat ribs anywhere else and I want to

93

eat them and not feel guilty about it. I don't want it to be my Joy Eat because I've already planned for ice cream with the kids on Sunday.

3. Action Plan
   The party is at 5, I will stick to my normal protocol for the day then at the dinner I will skip appetizers because I am saving up to really enjoy the ribs. I'll have up to 5 of them, I will have 2 glasses of pinot noir (the good stuff that I bring!) and I'll eat whatever side veggies other people bring - I'm bringing a big green salad so I know I'll be able to have my ribs with that. I'll eat to a +5 or less on the hunger scale - I don't want to feel gross, I just want to enjoy them.

4. Consequences I am signing up for

I may have sugar cravings the next day based on all that sauce. The scale may be up a pound or two based on the sugar and wine. My joints will probably be stiff in the morning (not sure why, but they seem to be when I eat off protocol lately.) I will want to keep eating other off protocol things when I am done with the ribs and two glasses of wine because that is how it works.

Step Six:

Putting it all Together: Travel with Ease

In this section I explain how all the things you've been working on at home – Steps 1-5 - can work for you when you're traveling too, and I also share my own positive experiences with Fat Fasting.

As a busy professional, you've got the double job of not only figuring out how to eat to lose weight at home with all its familiar habits and built-in temptation, but you also have to know how to tackle these other obstacles while traveling and living out of hotel rooms. You know it's not impossible, but it's been so hard in the past to make anything work - that's why you're here! You fly, hotel, convention, meet, happy hour, late-night dine after landing, and that's definitely part of the reason most diet plans don't work for you. You don't want to take the time to accurately count calories, prepare and portion food, keep things in a fridge, or pack a cooler so you can eat on "the plan." You need something that works for any stop along the way. This is it.

Change your Programming

I don't think many of us realize the depth of the unconscious programming we have around food - especially when we travel or eat with people we love. As you work through the steps I've presented here, it's very likely this will come up.

Be real and honest with yourself when you eat things that aren't on protocol or aren't a part of your plan that you made in advance. Usually it is because you either want to feel something (excitement, relief, indulgence, energy) or don't want to feel something (discomfort, bored, distracted, tired). It's not food's job to entertain you or support you emotionally. That's your job. Food is here to fuel you and yes, to be delicious and to satisfy, but not everything every time.

Just like the screwdriver is a crappy hammer and doesn't help when you need a wrench - food is not the answer to all your problems. That is the good news and the bad news. If you've been using food as your release valve, your entertainment section, your pleasure center, and your major distracter then you still have work to do. You have to figure out how to do life without relying on food as your tool for everything. Your solution for every problem. We all have been there - looking more forward to the food on the trip than the people we're hanging with – but what if the people were better than the food? The goal here is to for you to be comfortable in your body and in your life - even on the road.

Order from any Menu

Start by opening the menu and finding the salad section. If something looks good, have that. Make sure the dressing is full fat, or get it with oil or mayo. If the salad doesn't come with enough fat in it to satisfy you, ask the waiter to add avocado, bacon, or egg.

If you're not feeling their salad options ask for a burger or a sandwich, but have it with greens instead of the bread, bun, or roll. Remember, the goal here is fiber-rich vegetables paired with satisfying fat. Be creative! One of my clients, when she finds herself out with a group who has ordered pizzas to share, will slide the toppings off her crust and onto a salad. She gets to enjoy the part she likes best of pizza, and doesn't have that heavy, gross feeling from eating all that dough (and she's staying on protocol and continuing to lose weight!).

When looking over a menu, watch out for sweet sauces, ketchup, or sticky meat marinades that are mostly sugar. Do your best, be skeptical when you need to be, but don't freak out when things don't work out the best way for your protocol. I used to be a restaurant manager, and I can tell you that we liked helping people figure out how they can enjoy our food. So ask questions about the menu and have the server help you create a good option. They've often eaten there so much they know exactly what will work and taste great.

Alcohol

I lost all my weight while continuing to drink a few times a week. I probably could have lost weight faster if I drank less or not at all, but it was a part of my life, and I wanted to make weight loss work IN my life - not in spite of it.

Drinks are the same as food when it comes to your protocol - you want to plan them in advance. So, if you know that you're going out to dinner with coworkers tomorrow night and you want to enjoy a few glasses of wine - plan that today. If you don't end up drinking two, you just have one - fine. If you think you might have three, but only plan for two - hold up. Make the plan for three so that you have have the best chance at keeping your word to yourself.

It's just like with food, you want to do what you say you'll do. Make the plan have a little wiggle room in it just in case you need it. It doesn't hurt you NOT to drink the third glass but it does hurt you to drink the third glass having only planned to drink two. This all goes back to shedding old habits and fostering those new pathways you are creating in your brain by keeping your word to

I Wanted It

yourself.

Fat Fasting

The notion of fasting can really freak people out, and I strategically put this at the back of the book in hopes that by the time you got to this part – after working through the earlier steps to recognize old habits and become fat-adapted - you'd be ready for it. Fat Fasting is a valuable tool for weight loss and overall health, and an excellent tool for travelers.

Background

Your body LOVES homeostasis - it likes to keep things the same. One way this works against us in weight loss is that our bodies will work really hard to stay the same weight - no matter what we try. Intermittent fasting offers enough of a change from your body's normal routine that it shifts you into a different gear.

There are a lot of different processes in your body that can occur either faster or better when you shake it up in this way, giving your body a break from doing the work of processing your food.

Think about the fast you do every day already.

Yes, they call it breakfast for a reason break(the)fast. You fasted from the last thing you ate last night until the first thing you ate this morning so you know you can do this, it won't kill you. It's essential before doing a Fat Fast that you've worked through the earlier steps of this program and are fat-adapted. You'll still want to listen to your body before you try this. If you're really hungry that might not be the day for a fast and you should eat. You'll know when a Fat Fast makes sense for you because that choice will feel like the right or obvious next step.

This challenges a few ideas that we have been sold: Breakfast jump-starts your metabolism, you need breakfast as part of a healthy lifestyle, six small meals a day will keep your metabolism going...

No, no, and no. Your metabolism doesn't care if you eat breakfast! It has surprised me, as a former, avid, breakfast eater, that there really are people who don't like breakfast - I thought those were just dieters trying to look good. Nope, there are humans who would rather not eat until later in the day who are being shamed by conventional wisdom, who are eating when they are not hungry, who are gaining weight thinking they are doing what is "healthy."

If you're not hungry, don't eat. Even if the FDA or your mother tells you to. Your body is smart. It will take good care of you. You do not need to get your big human brain in the way and try to overthink this. Hunger is a sensation, and your body will signal your brain when it needs fuel. (There may be things getting in the way of the signal: Habit, hormones, etc.), but if you are a healthy the messaging system works. Trust it.

Fat Fasting doesn't mean you don't eat all day long, it means that what you do eat is high in fat. Eating things like nuts, an avocado, or maybe an egg, will help keep your blood sugar regulated (as compared to the popular juice diets that will spike your insulin), while still keeping your body in its fat-burning mode.

Fat Fasting for the Traveler

Before I became fat-adapted (before I even knew what that was), I took a trip to Sacramento and lived out of a hotel for a week. My daily diet looked similar to this every day: Grab a green juice and a black coffee for the morning round of meetings. Eat the egg and toast or oatmeal from the continental breakfast, grab a banana for later in case I got hungry - hungry or not, I always ate it, it's a banana, it's healthy! Between breakfast and lunch, there was trail mix and I usually had some at the mid-morning break. There were M&M's in there, and they were the motivator to eat the rest of what they bothered to throw in with the chocolate. At lunch time I'd go find a sandwich somewhere, maybe on a few of the days it was a salad. Back in for the afternoon and I was back in the trail mix. Then it was mid-afternoon break when I could grab a cookie that the hotel made fresh every afternoon. They weren't bad - they weren't great either - but they were there, melty, and free... Back in the meeting to make it through the rest of the day.

Dinner was out and it was Mexican, a burger, or Thai food. A few nights, I grabbed frozen yogurt on my way back from dinner, did a little work in my hotel room, and went to bed. On the flight home, I remember a frantic hunt for food because I was genuinely scared of being hungry on the plane. I ran around buying snacks I didn't need just to stave off that fear. I was so hung up on the what, the when, and the how of eating - and that was the norm!

Flash forward to my flight last Thursday. I was up at 4:30 am and in the air at 6:10. At Seatac, I got a grande Americano with heavy cream so I could work on my computer until the flight boarded for Dulles at 9:00. I grabbed a bag of cashews and a water from the newsstand and got on the plane. I'd been up 4.5 hours and I was calm. I was at a zero or +1 on the hunger scale. I boarded a five or so hour flight and all I had were nuts - and no plan to eat plane food. I was sustained by the fat in my coffee and off my body and I really enjoyed not caring, not hurrying, and not having to figure out how to eat a meal on that tiny tray.

Mid-way through the flight, I had a handful of cashews when my hunger level got to about a -2. I noticed about 10 minutes later I was still at what felt like a -2 so I ate another handful and called it good. I wanted to be sure I didn't get overly hungry while Fat Fasting, but honestly, I was totally fine, I could have done without the second handful. On arrival I had a 30-minute cab ride, a few hours of catching up with folks and getting dinner ordered, and it was 9 pm before I ate and I was at a -3 on the Hunger Scale.

Did you feel how much extra time I had in that travel day? I wasn't waiting for service at restaurants, I wasn't deciding where to eat, what to eat, if I had time. I didn't have to waste time or willpower making those decisions. I eliminated a lot of brain chatter (to cupcake or not to cupcake is *not* the question), wasted time, and bought food I didn't even need to eat. It's an added stress and travel has enough stressors.

For me, Fat Fasting on travel days has made them so much more enjoyable. I have fun choosing how I want to spend my time, and I feel so much calmer. I know that I won't starve to death during my flight; my body is fat-adapted so I no longer have the head-achy crashes that happen when you're used to running on cheap, sugar-filled fuel. If I'm hungry, I eat nuts or something high in fat. Then I check in with myself again to see where I'm at on the hunger scale.

Trip Plan

My client Mary just recently went to visit a friend for the weekend. She was nervous because she is new to all of this, and the norm is go to her friend's and overeat and over-drink all weekend. She didn't want to hurt her friend's feelings, feel deprived, or have even more discomfort socially than she normally does. I want to share this because I think it will surprise you how much leeway Mary gave herself when making her plan.

We are so used to planning for what we think we 'should' do that, when the time comes, we go way off-plan and end up feeling guilty and frustrated – sometimes perpetuating a self-destructive cycle. Let's break that cycle. If you're here what you've been doing isn't working, so stick with me and try something new. For Mary, we wanted to create a plan that built in the overeating (eating more than she needed for fuel) and over-drinking (planning to buffer her social anxiety), so that she can be honest with herself and more easily return to eating on protocol.

She knew she'd be showing up at 5 pm, and dinner would be hosted by her friend. It was also Mary's birthday, and she knew her friend would be spending hours making a cake, so she knew she would eat it – hungry or not - because she would want to honor her friend's hard work. Decision made in advance, no need for Mary to debate in the moment.

Mary knew that on arrival there would be appetizers and drinks. She didn't know the exact menu, but she could make an educated guess. People, including her friends, are pretty predictable. Just like me, if you ever come to my house there will be a home-brewed IPA on tap, and I'll serve wine, carrots, hummus, chips, salsa, cheeses and crackers and maybe an additional vegetable will be cut up. Life just isn't as unpredictable as we give it credit for.

Mary planned to have seven chips with whatever dip was there. Two bites of every kind of cheese. No more than six glasses of wine over the course of the evening. Sparkling water throughout the night. The friend would serve a protein and a few salads with beans or grains - as she always does. Mary planned on having a serving of each. Then cake and coffee - she knew she'd be overfull, but it was in the plan. If she wants it - she has it. No guilt, no questions. It's all in her plan.

Trip Plan

Date and Destination:

1. How do I want to feel when I get back home? What must I do on this trip to accomplish that goal?
2. What will be challenging about that?
3. In what ways will I try not to follow this plan?
4. Pick 3-5 situations I think will be challenging, visualize myself following through with the plan even when it is hard. Write them out here:
5. What did I wish I had planned better on my last trip?

Plan for travel day there:

What will I eat? Does this plan require that I bring anything with me? What else can I do to support this plan?

Plan for Travel day home:

What will I eat? Does my plan require me to bring anything with me? What else can I do prior to leaving to support this plan?

Trip Plan Example

Date and Destination:

In-Laws for Christmas.

How do I want to feel when I get back home?

I want to feel rested, filled, warm. I want to feel like it was a nourishing trip rather than a burn-the-candle-at-both-ends kind of trip (is that possible with a toddler?!)

What must I do on this trip to accomplish that goal?

Go to sleep at night instead of staying up too late drinking too much. Hot tub during the day when my daughter naps instead of late night. Do my morning practice before I go downstairs in the morning - otherwise it won't get done. Take a few naps while I'm there - two would probably do it. Drinking water would help too, I don't like the taste of the water there so I'm going to grab a few cases of sparkling water when I arrive because I can't NOT drink that stuff!

Plan my food and my alcohol the day before. Go for a walk each day and connect with individuals any chance I get.

In what ways will I try to not follow this plan?

The habit for me is to get more and more tired when I travel and then do less and less of what I know works for me! I'll be "too tired" to self-coach or plan or meditate - but I'm doing it anyway because I will feel great because of it. I think *normalizing that the things that are good for me ARE the uncomfortable things sometimes is good. It doesn't always feel EASY to do the thing that's good for me.*

Pick 3-5 situations I think will be challenging. Visualize following through with the plan even when it is hard. Write them out here:

1. *First night I arrive, we'll all be excited, a little road weary, and ready for that good Sonoma County wine. I'll plan ahead to eat whatever is served that is on protocol for Dinner. Not snack - even if it is foods that are on my protocol. 3 glasses of wine or less throughout that night and go to bed by 10.*

2. *Christmas Eve Dinner: My brother-in-law is cooking so I'm sure there will be protocol foods*

Caryn Gillen

to eat so I'll plan for that - but he is also serving Manhattans - and I know I have a harder time doing what I said I'd do when I drink so I want to be sure and set a very clear plan on the 23rd so it's a no brainer. I just want to enjoy myself and not have any chatter about food etc.

3. Christmas Day. I love Bulletproof coffee, I've never done it at their house but I'm going to this trip - it's the thing that keeps me feeling good until noon so I don't get distracted by the lounge around and overeat tradition that is Christmas!

Plan for travel day there:

Bulletproof coffee in the morning. Fat Fast on the place until Dinner - then protocol dinner with no more than 3 *glasses of wine.*

Plan for Travel day home:

Bulletproof coffee in the morning. Fat Fast on the plane until protocol dinner at home. I won't have any food in the house so I'll plan to pick up lettuce wrapped burgers on the way home. No fries as I'm sure I'll have had enough rich food by then!

Caryn Gillen

Chapter 4: Obstacles

The easiest way I know of to tackle hard situations is to approach them with curiosity, rather than judgment. There will be times in this process that you will be derailed, that you will go off-protocol, that you will fall into old habits. That's okay, that's normal. You may feel shame and guilt, and that's normal too, the key is to not let those emotions prevent you from doing the work. In this chapter I've presented four frequently-encountered obstacles, and practical worksheets to help you work through them. The trick here is to be onto ourselves, while also being kind to ourselves. We want to learn from our mistakes, not punish ourselves for making them.

Obstacle One: Overeating/Going off-Protocol

This exercise is a great way to take a step back when you've over-eaten. The goal here is to learn from our mistakes and move on without guilt.

Write It Down and Move On:

1. What did you overeat that wasn't on protocol?
2. Why did you overeat? Be very specific.
3. What did you notice?
4. What would've worked better? What else could you have done?
5. What did you learn?
6. How can you let this go now?
7. How do you want to feel about this moving forward?
8. How will you handle this next time?

Example:
1. What did you overeat that wasn't on protocol?
Chocolate Cake.

2. Why did you overeat? Be very specific.
I wanted it. It looked good. I'm

never around this bakery so I wanted to take advantage. I wanted to taste it. I've walked a ton today. I wanted to be filled up.

3. What did you notice?
I noticed it wasn't as good as I wanted it to be. I wished it was better. I didn't feel that good after it. I always feel like it's not worth it in the middle of it - but I finish it anyway. How come I don't remember that before I start eating it?

4. What would've worked better? What else could you have done?
I could have decided my next Joy Eat would be chocolate cake - even if it wasn't from this bakery. I could have done a thought download about it and probably

realized I was actually just tired and cake can't help tired. I could have had a few squares of dark chocolate and been done with it.

5. What did you learn?
   I learned that food is just food. It never does the job of taking care of me.

6. How can you let this go now?
   I can let this go because I am going to remember this - and learn from it. Next time I want to overeat or eat off protocol I want to ask myself "Why?" And keep asking it until I get to the heart of it.

7. How do you want to feel about this moving forward?
   Moving forward I want to feel kind towards myself for thinking

it would make me feel good - but also onto myself that I knew deep down it wouldn't. I could have taken good care of me but I chose to check out from life and I used the chocolate cake to do it. I tried to pretend I had good reasons - I didn't.

8. How will you handle this next time?
   Next time I'll ask myself why, and I'll take the time to get to the bottom of it before I make another move. If I can't be at least that thoughtful with myself then I can be sure I'm not eating for the reasons I want to.

Obstacle Two: Losing Motivation/Falling off the Wagon

This is the worksheet you use when you are feeling down because the scale isn't moving fast enough, or you don't think this is working, or maybe you "fell off the wagon" in some way or another and you're just not as into it as you want to be.

How to get from "Checked out" to "Checked in"

1. Why did I check out?
2. Where am I right now, what am I doing that is "checked out?"
3. If this is the turning point, what do I want the results of checking back in to be?
4. What, if anything, is stopping this from happening?
5. What tools will I use to keep moving toward my goals?
6. What else do I need to know to let go and move forward?

Example:

1. Why did I check out?

> I stopped doing what works for me. Once I did that it was a pretty easy slide right off! Why did I do that...? I think I got too comfortable. I often have the thought "I can get away with it." In one form or another and it does NOT serve me.

2. Where am I right now, what am I doing that is "checked out"?

> I'm using food to distract me from what is important. I keep feeling restless and then eating over that. Totally what I used to do. I keep thinking I just need to re-do my plan and get reinvigorated - but in reality I just need to do what works - every day. Every. Day.

3. If this is the turning point, what do I want the results of checking back in to be?

> *Goal weight. More free time where I'm not hiding from life/thinking about food. If I really turned it around today I would stop right now and plan for tomorrow and be done with it. Decision made - as good as done.*

4. What, if anything, is stopping me from making that happen?

> *Nothing. I'll think my brain is - but let's be honest. Nothing is stopping me.*

5. What tools will I use to keep moving toward my goals?

> *Food journal, weigh everyday, self-coaching, planning one day*

ahead. Taking massive action (not just consuming information but putting it into practice.).

6. What else do I need to know or let go of to move forward?

I know that I've got this, I have everything I need, I don't need to make it more complicated - I need to keep it simple!

Obstacle Three: Outside Expectations

"The bartender gave me a free shot so I had to take it." "I love her pie, she makes it just for me so I had to have a piece." "Everyone was celebrating, I had to join in." "It was their birthday so I had cake." "Your example here..."

Treats happen. Life happens. Holidays happen. Birthdays happen. They are not hard or easy - they just are. It's your thoughts about them and what will make others happy, or what you 'should' do that you need to figure out. The good news is that all these things happen every year - people will be offering you good things in happy, sad, or even boring situations all the time. So let's just decide now how you're going to respond.

You do not need to eat anything that anyone gives you. Ever. You can choose to, or you can choose not to, but let's be clear: YOU get to choose. Food doesn't happen to you. So, what can you do? I see two options:

1. Expect it and plan to have it or not. (You could use Joy Eat or the Exception Plan worksheet if you want to plan it.)
2. Don't eat it.

I know, it's all so clear on paper - but in your head it's all fuzzy and feels hard or confusing. That's why the planning is essential. Every time.

I was thinking about this the other day - if you let other people's events, celebrations, and "expectations" for your eating rule how you eat you'll never get anywhere! For one, these things are happening ALL THE TIME. There'd never be a good time to start dieting or to eat on protocol. My second thought was how crazy it is to allow someone else to decide what you should eat or why or when!

Just because they prepared it and liked it and wanted to have "party food" or whatever doesn't mean that has anything to do with me or my meal plan or my goals or what I like. Why would I ever let someone else dictate my fuel? I drive a diesel car, I would never drive it up to a gas station and have the attendant serve up gasoline because it's his birthday. I order diesel 100% of the time because that's the best fuel for my car.

What if we were that clear about food?
- [ ] Be clear about the results you are creating – refer back to the letter from your future

self you wrote in Chapter 3, or write another one - make them compelling enough that no cookie can break them down!

☐ Plan for things you want to make exceptions for a day ahead (use the tools provided in this book.)

☐ Stick to your plan even when unexpected things come up, even when it's uncomfortable (that is the affirmation that you're doing it right!).

Obstacle Four: Fear of Failure

In weight loss we often feel uncomfortable because we are changing – that discomfort is how you know you're doing it right. That discomfort can feel overwhelming, and when it does I want you to hone in on the good part of the change that is coming. The best way to do that is to sit down and dump your thoughts on paper - I like to use questions like the ones that follow to really dig in and coach myself. Try using these - but don't stop there - if you find yourself going in another direction or getting off topic - go with it.

Self Coaching Prompts

1. What is the uncomfortable situation?
2. What is the primary feeling here?
3. What skill am I developing by being willing to feel this discomfort?
4. What do I risk missing out on by not being willing to feel this discomfort?
5. How can my future self's perspective help me right now?
6. What is my plan for taking this learning forward?

Example:

1. What is the uncomfortable situation?

> I'm up 6 pounds from goal weight. I am a little weirded out that I was okay with it until now. I just kept thinking "It's okay, I'll just lose it." I will - but, like, when?!

2. What is the primary feeling here?

> Nervous. Like, what the heck, I can't be a weight loss coach and be sloppy with myself!

3. What skill am I developing by being willing to feel this discomfort?

> The skill of being onto myself, honest, of telling myself the truth and not justifying. It's so easy and comforting to think, "It's okay, I'll just lose it. It's just two pounds." It's

funny because I should KNOW as soon as one of those little high-pitched thoughts comes up that I am hiding from myself. What do I risk missing out on by not being willing to feel this discomfort?

4. What do I risk missing out on by not being willing to feel this discomfort?

If I really played this out I could let it take me out; I could make it mean that I'm not meant to do this, that I shouldn't do what I do. I would miss out on the strengthening of my commitment, learning I can come back from here and it doesn't have to be a big deal, I just do what I know works.

5. How can my future self's perspective help me right now?

She reminds me we've done this

before - and that if I'm focused on the weight I'm doing it wrong! She knows that every time I focus on the scale I gain weight - it's because when I do that I'm hoping, and hoping doesn't get me anywhere! I have to focus on creating MY LIFE and the scale will fall in line. She nails it, every time. Every. Damn. Time.

6. What is your plan for taking this learning forward?

Do what I know works. The things that got me to goal weight worked - and I've given them up and freaked myself out. So now I have to do the work of making them a priority again and the rest will resolve itself. So, getting up at 5:30 so I can have my morning practice of self-coaching and meditation. I'll be packing my lunch and making the coffee the night before and planning and writing tomorrow's food in my Food Journal today.

Chapter 5: Conclusion

We've talked about how conventional wisdom is keeping you fat and what you can do instead so you can actually lose weight. I've shared the tools you need to keep you on track while you are losing weight - both at home and on the road.

These are the tools that work for me and for my clients. You've also tapped into the vision of your future self, you at goal weight, and you can use that connection to help pull you towards the results you're creating.

Right now you're overweight and you're uncomfortable in your clothes and maybe even in your life. You're ready to lose weight but too busy to do anything that won't work and you're understandably leery because dieting has failed you.

I want you to enjoy your time at home more because you know what your plan is with your food. To have the peace of mind that the way you are eating is moving you towards the results you want. I hope my Six-Step Process will help you enjoy the travel more, knowing that no matter what situation life and work throw at you you've got it nailed.

You know what it takes to get there. It's not easy but it is doable - especially with commitment and support. Now ask yourself how your life would be different if you had this outcome? If you knew you could travel for work with ease and not gain weight - even lose it.

My wish for you is that you are able to lead the busy and successful life you've created for yourself - even on the road - and lose weight. I want you to come home, toss your suitcase in the corner and get on with your day and your life feeling confident that you've got this. You know what you are doing when you leave and you've got yourself set up when you get home. That is everything.

That's why we're all losing weight; not for some magic number on a scale, but to get to the land where our future self lives. She gardens, swims more at the beach, actually rides the road bike she bought - she lives her life – and starting today, you can too.

Next Steps:

From here you have some options, you can:

a. Do nothing and stay the same.
b. Implement some or all of the tools on your own.
c. Come work with me.

If you chose A or B your next steps are:

1. Go to www.caryngillen.com and sign up to get weekly communication from me along with other special offers that only go out to my list. If you have any questions I'm here to help and I'd love to hear from you.

2. Get to work.

If you chose option C:

1. Go to www.caryngillen.com/work-with-me to apply to work with me. Once that

application comes in we'll schedule your 20-minute, free, no obligation, consult.

2. At our scheduled appointment time we'll have a few minutes to check in and answer any initial questions you may have. Do a little coaching on one topic of your choosing.

3. You'll either decide you're ready to get to work while we are on the phone or you may take some time to think about it. Either way, I'll follow-up via email and we'll go from there. If either of us don't think we are a good fit to work together you'll still have all these tools and you can go back and decide on option A or B.

If this book spoke to you I hope you'll take these next steps and reach out.

Thank you,

Caryn

Caryn Gillen

Acknowledgements

Thank you to all the clients I've had to date and to those of you yet to come. You continue to help me grow and fine tune the work that is this book. It's one thing to have my own experience and to read books that support my work but to have been trusted with your weight loss journey continues to be a great honor. Thank you for saying yes to you, your courage fills my heart and knocks me off my feet regularly.

To the people who helped bring this book from idea to paperback - thank you. Angela Lauria, I've wanted to work with you since I started coaching years ago, I was right all along, thank you! Katie Bennett, without you this would not be a book. Thank you for sharing your gifts so that I can share mine. I am forever grateful to you. Angie Beauchaine, you wrote a foreward that made me want to sit down and reread my own book! Thank you for sharing your experience and expertise with us.

To my sweet family, thank you for giving me time and space to write, re-write, edit, proof, and print. It was no small feat for any of us and I am so thankful for the opportunity.

To my chosen teachers, Brooke Castillo and Evelyn Tribole, I would not be where I am without you having gone first. Thank you for sharing and inspiring, for teaching and coaching, and for offering a new way to those who have struggled.

Finally, to you, dear reader, thank you. I wrote this book for you, I wrote it with the hope that you may struggle one day less, so that you may lose the first five pounds or the last five (or both!) and do it with the knowing that you've found the magic bullet - and it was always you. You've got this, you have everything you need.

Trust it.

About the Author

Caryn Gillen, M.A., is a Life Coach who lives in Eugene, Oregon with her husband Todd and daughter Liv. She works with clients to improve their quality of life, with a special emphasis on health and wellness for the busy professional. You can learn more about Caryn and her work at www.caryngillen.com.

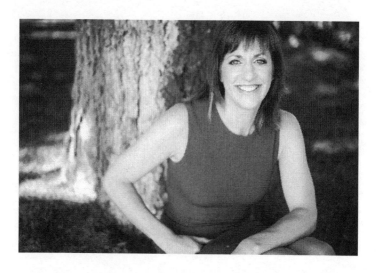

Thank You

Thank you for reading this book for being willing to even consider the possibility of becoming that future you, the one who travels with ease and comes home lighter. I wish you the very best wherever your travels may take you.

Caryn

www.caryngillen.com

Made in the USA
San Bernardino, CA
20 January 2018